A Bedside Manner

The art of elegant consulting

By Dr Mark Chambers

A bedside manner

ISBN: 978-0995459991

Published by Ann Jaloba Publishing, Sheffield S10 2QH

Note to Readers

The information, including opinion and analysis contained herein are based on the author's personal experiences. The information provided herein should not be used for diagnosing or treating a health problem or disease. Readers are advised to consult a doctor for medical advice. The author and the publisher make no warranties, either expressed or implied, concerning the accuracy, applicability, activeness, reliability or suitability of the contents. If you wish to apply or follow the advice or recommendations mentioned herein, you take full responsibility for your actions. The author and the publisher of this book shall in no event be held liable for any direct, indirect, incidental or other consequential damages arising directly or indirectly from any use of the information contained in this book. All content is for information only and is not warranted for content accuracy or any other implied or explicit purpose.

Dedication

This book is a summary of what I have learned in 32 years as a GP, Practitioner and Trainer. It is dedicated to my readers with the request that you take whatever resonates with you from this and improve on it.

We all learn most from those around us, our teachers, those we read and those we work with and for. This book is heavily indebted to the thoughts, insights, writings and teachings of many who have crossed my path in my professional life. Some are very well-known, others work more quietly under the radar. I would like to acknowledge all their contributions to my thoughts and practice and therefore to this book.

A bedside manner

Contents

A bedside manner

INTRODUCTION

"If I have seen further than others, it is by standing on the shoulders of giants"

Isaac Newton

Have you noticed, either as a doctor or as a patient, how some consultations appear to just run smoothly, and others just do not flow? This book aims to help you identify the factors that govern this: how to identify the difference that makes the difference. This is in the hope that by gaining these insights the practice of consulting, the cornerstone of the practice of medicine, can be increasingly elegant, enjoyable and effective for all concerned. These are essential communication skills, with applicability well beyond just the particular context of the GP consultation.

My intention in writing this book is to present what I have learned in over 30 years of learning, practising and teaching The Consultation. Over this time, I have developed a personal style that stands the test of time and continues to work well for me. I invite my readers to cherry-pick from the ideas that I present, and incorporate the bits which appeal into their work, so they can reasonably expect to continue to develop and adapt their consulting style to deliver consistently the best possible outcomes and enjoy the process.

A bedside manner

I first read the quotation at the beginning of this section on a plaque on the wall outside the library in The Royal Society of Medicine in London, while staying there when studying for the Post-Graduate Diploma in Medical Hypnosis which I completed in 2012. It resonated with me. Although some of what is to follow I have developed for myself, much of what I have learned has, inevitably, been passed down to me by the many excellent teachers I have studied with and modelled over the years. Where I am aware of the source, I have acknowledged this in the text. If anyone recognises something I have said as originating from them I hope they will contact me so I can make sure this is duly acknowledged in any future work. I would also welcome any feedback.

I want to start out by expressing my gratitude to all my teachers for sharing their wisdom, knowledge and skills. When I took my Hippocratic Oath on qualifying as a doctor in Sheffield in 1981, this included the obligation, in due course, to pass on what I had learned to the next generation. I am happy, in my turn, to share the approaches that have helped me to a very satisfying career in General Practice. The bulk of it I have assimilated from the instruction and models of those who have taught me.

The roots of this work can be found in a conversation I had with a good friend and mentor on the golf course in 2009. The message I received from him is that everyone has a book in them, and that my 30 years' experience as a GP and Trainer, and my interest in complementary methods, meant that what I have to share is unique and may well be useful to a wide audience. Since that conversation I have made notes from time to time when something struck me as potentially worthy of sharing. These notes have become the basis of this book.

Introduction

My background

I consider myself extremely fortunate to have had a career in General Practice. My father was a GP in rural Lincolnshire, and I knew from a very early age that I wanted to do what my Dad did. He was a smoker and died as a consequence, prematurely, in 2002. Since his death, from time to time, when faced with a tricky problem, I still find myself asking what he would do in that situation. The answer usually comes to me, often after a night's sleep.

I suspect it was my father who first stimulated my interest in hypnosis. I was away at boarding school from the age of 10, and initially very unhappy. This affected my sleep. I remember my father teaching me a progressive relaxation technique that I found helpful. This taught me an important lesson, which has under-pinned my approach to my professional work. Every patient, myself included, has the resources within themselves to deal with whatever life throws at them.

At school I enjoyed Latin. The vocabulary has proved helpful with understanding and using medical terminology, and the attention to detail in the grammar has left me with an abiding pedantry for accurate use of language.

The word 'doctor' has particular relevance to me. I was privileged to be a GP trainer for 24 years. One of the first questions I asked a trainee GP joining me is what they understood by the term: 'doctor'. This was usually greeted with a stunned silence, followed by a variation along the lines of diagnosing and treating disease. For me this is incomplete. The origin of the word 'doctor' is Latin. It means 'teacher'. My take on this is that the doctor's role is to assist the patient in their life-long task of learning to take good care of themselves, and particularly in the skills of making better choices and decisions. Much of this takes place within the context of their 'disease', but, for me, the doctor's responsibility often goes far beyond this, into all facets of that individual's experience. This is particularly so in the General Practice context. This book addresses the aspect of teaching in the role of the doctor. This means seeing the patient, not as being broken and in need of fixing, but from the point of view of a teacher. This involves identifying and addressing the learning needs of both teacher and learner. The essential, ancient principle is that the body keeps the score. When things happen to us and around us, our body, via our senses, assimilates the information. This information comes into consciousness initially as feelings and emotions. This is the principle of the Primacy of Affect. The body keeping the score. Our cognitive mind then produces a narrative that accounts for our experience, and we respond to that narrative as though it is true. If the stimulus is sufficiently powerful or prolonged, these messages develop into symptoms, as we experience disease. The body-mind has its own natural homeostatic and healing mechanisms. Hippocrates was referring to these when he said that it is natural forces within us that are the true healers of disease. The role of the professional in this model is to help optimise the conditions for these natural forces to do their work.

Introduction

The Context of General Practice : The meta-physician

For those looking for a book on evidence-based practice, please stop now. Evidence-based medicine has an essential place in the practicing habits of all health-care professionals. For me our responsibilities to our patients go well beyond this. In English General Practice we have the privilege of being the only professionals in the National Health Service who cannot discharge patients. We have a registered list of patients and it is our duty to help them find a way through whatever issues they choose to bring to us, all the way to the end. We have to keep going, with our patients, often long after the evidence-base is exhausted. Many years ago, in a National Census, in describing the GPs job, a colleague summarised the situation admirably and succinctly: "Anything, for anyone, anytime, anywhere." In my 36 years as a doctor I have yet to have a patient come and ask specifically for an evidence-based approach to their problems. Doubtless there is an assumption on their part that that is what they are getting. I suspect that a good proportion of what happens in the doctor-patient interaction is not evidence-based. It cannot be. Patients come back to the GP when the evidence-base has been thoroughly explored and deployed.

This book is much more concerned with the Art of the Practice of Medicine rather than the science. It addresses not so much what to do; there already exists a whole range of excellent books and other resources addressing this, but rather how to develop the context in which to efficiently and elegantly deliver our knowledge and skills so they can be most effective. This work aims to help the reader develop their own insights into the process of the Consultation and thus develop the attitudes, values, understandings and flexibility which will enhance their ability to interact effectively with their patients, to the greatest benefit of all concerned.

In my world a key life skill is asking better questions. In this circumstance, not so much "is it 'true'?", but "is it 'useful'?"   My patients come with their lists of problems, and do not want to be told that there is X% chance of a favourable outcome with this approach, unless X=100. They want a 100% result, for them. In my opinion we have a role as caring professionals to go beyond purely evidence-based interventions, and help our patients learn to make all the changes they need to give themselves the best chance of achieving the outcomes they seek. My approach to my professional work is that there is much that can be done to ensure that our patients find themselves in the group with the good outcome, when the statistics are analysed. In the early days of NLP, one of the original researchers, Judith Delozier, declared herself a 'searcher' rather than a 'researcher.' I understand the position. Each consultation with a patient is the starting of a new page. The situation is unique and has not existed before. The focus is not in the past, but in the present, with an eye to the future. There is only ever 'now'.

This is not to say that there is not much to learn from the past, but thankfully it is over, and there is a future to be created. Keep the useful patterns from the past, adapt those that warrant it to the current and future circumstances, evolve new patterns and discard the redundant ones, with due gratitude to them for what they have done. Travel light. This book addresses some of the processes involved in this. It is primarily concerned with process rather than content: not so much what to do: each individual practitioner develops their own unique style. This is about the process involved: how to do it. The attitudes, values and personal habits which generate success.

An important part of the NHS GP's function is as gatekeeper of the available NHS and Social Services. Knowing the limits of our personal expertise is key, and knowing how and where to refer patients on, when we do not have the tools to meet their needs, is an important part of the role. The responsibility does not rest there. If the outcome is favourable, so be it. If not, the patient returns. Eventually there comes a point, with some patients, where the apparent options have been exhausted. In my view Western Medicine tends to frame patients' issues as 'problems'. A cause is sought and usually external solutions deployed: medication, physical treatments, surgery and talking: 'getting it out'. These are often successful. When they have been exhausted, and the desired outcome not achieved, the professionals involved may advise the patient that they have done all they can and suggest they return to their GP. For the GP this leaves the option of accepting the status-quo and resigning the patient to their fate, or helping the patient explore avenues which have not so far been identified. This involves mobilising the innate resources the patient has, an approach more favoured in Eastern approaches to medicine, many of which predate Western, Hippocratic Medicine by centuries.

The Problem

Currently the National Health Service is facing major resource challenges. The junior doctors have been in dispute with the Government over modifications to their contract and morale is low. Every winter the system is stretched beyond capacity. We face a climate of increasing demand and dwindling resources.

Patients have greater access to information via the media than ever before and an increasing expectation that medicine has answers which did not previously exist. Often this is correct. Frequently not. While there is not a pill for every ill, new medical interventions are developing and appearing all the time, assisted by the ease of communication that modern technology provides for researchers. All this comes at a financial cost which the NHS administration and governments have to monitor and budget for. The current norm in English General Practice, is to work with a 10-minute appointment model, so effective use of time is at a premium.

All this is placing increasing stress on doctors and burnout is occurring. The idea of a work-life balance is much more prevalent among younger doctors, who are more aware of the importance of looking after their own health and well-being than previous generations of practitioners. Stress-related illness is prevalent in the medical profession. There is much that can be done, within current constraints, to address this, and integrate good working patterns into a fulfilling lifestyle. Currently doctors are increasingly retiring early, moving to other areas of medicine or emigrating to seek more favourable working conditions. I would like General Practice to find its way again, and once again become an enjoyable and rewarding career-option. The principles identified in this book are equally applicable in a much wider context. I hope there is something in here for anyone who consults.

Introduction

The Promise

I learned from reading Virginia Satir's teaching (Satir, 1988) that that the problem is not the problem. It is only a symptom of something much deeper. Coping is the challenge, and it is the way we cope that makes the difference.

In preparing this book I have reflected on all that I have learned and how I have developed my approach to consulting effectively and enjoyably as far as possible. I have sought to identify the elements which build a consulting style that is flexible, elegant, effective and ultimately, satisfying: the components of a successful consultation. The intention is to identify how I develop the best environment within which to generate results with and for patients, and make the process fun as far as possible. Elegance in this context is a term derived from computer science; achieving the desired outcome in as few steps as possible. For many of my readers this will be old wine in a new bottle. I present it in the hope that it will spur the reader to explore how to work at their best, build their confidence, and continue to evolve their most effective style, as they adapt to the ever-changing working environment and context. This in turn will help beat burnout, build resilience and kindle enjoyment in their work and an enduring enthusiasm for a career in General Practice.

There are many excellent books and sources of information available about the content of the GP Consultation. In this work I am addressing the process of effective consulting: not so much what to do, but how to do it. These are my ideas on how to deliver a successful consultation.

The Population

I have written this book primarily to support doctors who are in the early days of their exploration of General Practice. However, there is much in here which will be of interest to more experienced doctors who wish to reflect on the process of consultation in General Practice and develop more flexibility and adaptability to their consultation style. While my focus has been on what can be achieved in 10 minutes with a patient, the information is equally relevant to anyone who is interested in developing their consultation style in other contexts too.

The Solution

I explore many aspects of the consultation. These include the accessing of the states in the doctor and the patient most likely to generate good solutions, and the establishment and maintenance of rapport. Next comes building hope and motivation. Then effective methods of goal-setting, delivering, reflecting and learning are identified. The importance of developing useful habits and practising successful patterns of intervention is discussed, with the desired result of developing an elegant consulting style that generates the best results for patients and job-satisfaction for the doctor.

For ease of discussion I have isolated eight different components of effective interventions for discussion. In practice, several of these elements usually occur simultaneously, so this work is not intended as a 'walk-through' the consultation, but rather a dissection and examination of some of the more pertinent constituent parts.

Introduction

My intention is that, by application of the principles presented here, the doctor will be able to work comfortably, efficiently and elegantly within a ten-minute consultation model. By incorporating a reflective approach to their work, the reader will learn how to consistently improve and build fun and enjoyment into their professional life. I have incorporated ideas and principles from many of the complementary disciplines I have trained in; including several hypnosis methods, Neuro-Linguistic Programming, Mindfulness, Reiki and other Mind-Body Energy techniques.

For the sake of clarity, in many places I have been quite dogmatic. One of the skills I encourage is the formulation of good questions. I refer to my earlier point about asking better questions and would encourage the reader to read this book, not from the position of asking if what I am saying is true, but rather, is it useful?

Let us begin . . .

References

Satir V. (1988) *The New Peoplemaking* Science and Behaviour Books Inc Palo Alto CA USA ISBN 0-8314-0070-6

A bedside manner

CHAPTER 1 - Your State

In this chapter, I am going to offer a definition of 'state' as I use the concept in this book and explain why it is of great importance in all that follows. I will discuss how we generate our state and to what extent we can be voluntarily involved in this and how this knowledge can be effectively used in the consultation.

I recall a discussion that brought home to me just how crucial our state is to our experience, and how easily and quickly it can fluctuate. Changing just one word in a sentence can change vastly the meaning we give it and our individual response to what is being said. In an NLP training, one of my fellow students shared the insight that, in a successful consultation, the patient comes in in **A** right state and leaves in **THE** right state. It is hard to imagine a more succinct summation of what our work in the consulting room is about.

Towards a definition of State

Your state is the sum total of all your neuro-biological processing in the present moment: physiological, emotional, psychological, spiritual, and cognitive. Information comes into your nervous system from the external and internal world through your senses. This information is initially processed outside of consciousness and a tiny abstract of it is presented to your conscious mind as your awareness. You experience this as thoughts, feelings and emotions. The simultaneous, unconscious processing is reflected in your physiology: heart rate, respiratory pattern, posture, muscle tension and facial expression. All this adds up to your state. These experiences are then amalgamated to produce your behaviour. The whole process is automatic, and occurs most of the time without your conscious involvement. This is habit. Mostly, we run on habit and do not give this whole process any thought. This is essential for our survival and quality of life. If we had to learn anew how to open a door every time we encountered a door handle, life would be so slow we would never achieve anything of significance. The good news is that our state is itself largely a function of where we place our focus. If we choose to think about it, we do have choice about this, and can deliberately modulate our state.

This is important because state determines attitude, which in turn generates choices and the consequent results. Attitude is a metaphor from the science of avionics, meaning angle of approach. (Many terms in modern psychology are metaphors from established science, especially engineering, for example stress, strain and resilience.)

First things first, getting your state right

Stephen Covey, in his *Seven Habits of Highly Effective People* (Covey, 1989) identifies being pro-active and doing 'first things first' as the first two of these habits. Balint (Balint, 1964) identified the concept of the 'drug doctor'. This echoes Hippocrates who identified the relationship between the physician and his patient as key in the outcome of the interaction. In any enterprise or activity in life, the single most important factor in generating the outcome that emerges is your state. Get this right first then get on and do whatever you wish to do.As well as being key to our outcome, state is also a vital interventional tool. States are contagious. We are all aware of how the arrival of a new person in a room or group can dramatically affect the dynamics of the group and the mood of the room. These people may be thought of as Radiators and Drains. Some people lighten up the atmosphere simply by being there, others seem to sap the vitality and energy from the gathering. All this happens before any words are exchanged.

Parallel Processing

One of the themes of this book is parallel processing. If you want someone to go somewhere, you have to go there yourself first. If you are stressed, bored and uninterested, the patient will pick up on this before any verbal communication has taken place. As discussed in the introduction, the body keeps the score. Our first response is emotional and manifests physically: it is felt in the body. State is communicated at this pre-linguistic level.

Initial communication is made at a pre-verbal level and this is key to developing an effective professional relationship. Our first response to meeting a new situation is at an affective, emotional level. This occurs within nano-seconds and long before we have developed a linguistic representation in our internal dialogue, let alone formulated it in any external, verbal expression. The order of events is feel/emote, *then* possibly think, then behave. Accessing resourceful states in ourselves is a skill that can be learned and practised. It is my contention that this is an essential skill for generating elegance in consulting.

The Doctor as Teacher

In my introduction, I discussed the concept of the doctor as a teacher. Developing this idea, one of the teacher's roles is to help the student identify their unique learning needs. These are also the learning needs of the doctor, in the context of the GP consultation. The doctor needs to make sense of all the information the patient is communicating, verbally and, most important, non-verbally. The doctor also needs to be aware of what is *not* being said. From this the doctor can develop an understanding of the meaning that this information has. This will, of course, be different for the doctor and the patient. It is here that the root of effective intervention lies. Both doctor and patient are sorting information (we call this parallel-processing) simultaneously and generating unique meanings and possibilities.

For the doctor to do this most effectively, an optimum learning state is essential. The best learners are young children. When learning they are curious, adventurous, non-critical, non-judgmental, playful, experimental and often fearless. All this contributes to their creativity. This uses their amazing powers of imagination, unfettered by any critical faculty (this remains dormant until around the age of seven years). Bringing this creative curiosity to the Consultation and finding the sweet-spot between the known and the unknown is an excellent starting point for generating a satisfactory encounter.

This willingness to approach every consultation as a new opportunity, with an attitude of creative curiosity, is something that has been highlighted for me from reading and training with Dr. Stephen Gilligan. Early in his career Dr. Gilligan studied with Dr. Milton Erickson, and has subsequently continued to evolve his own Generative approach to therapy, coaching, personal growth and life. Dr. Erickson was an extraordinary psychiatrist who developed his own unique and highly effective communication and linguistic style, based around his life-experiences and also his phenomenal professional knowledge and experience in the fields of psychiatry and hypnosis. His work has informed much of what is effective in modern psychotherapy and also in interpersonal communication in many fields. It has informed much of what is to follow in these pages. I will say more about the optimum learning state in Chapter 7, on Delivering.

The single most important gift we can ever give to anyone, in the Consultation and anywhere else, is the quality of our attention. To give our patients our best attention we have to empty our mind of pre-judgements and everything else, and to be open to their world, with an attitude of non-judgmental acceptance and creative curiosity. This is the key to generating success. This need only be for a very few moments in a consultation. The more flexible we are in adjusting our state appropriately, the better will we be able to address ourselves most fruitfully to our consulting.

None of this is new thinking. This awareness has informed teaching since ancient times. Epicetus, writing in the 1st Century AD said: "Men are disturbed, not by things, but by the principles and notions which they form concerning things." It is not what happens to you, but how you react to it that matters.

Victor Frankl (Frankl, 1959) sums up the importance of the awareness that we can choose our response, our state: "Between stimulus and response there is a space. In that space there is our power to choose our response. In our response lies our growth and our freedom. When we can no longer change a situation, we are challenged to change ourselves."

There are echoes of this same concept in many disciplines. In NLP John Grinder refers to the "know-nothing state," (Grinder, 2001). The "paying attention" of Mindfulness (Hanh, 2008). Csikszentmihalyi's Flow (Csikszentmihalyi, 1992) and the silent prayer which is part of many religious practices. Attaining this state is something which can be practised and mastered so that it can be produced at will. It can become independent of external factors.

Wherever we go we take ourselves with us. The ability and flexibility to generate appropriate, resourceful states is a key life-skill with applications way beyond the consulting room.

How to do it?

To prepare yourself to be your best in the consulting room, to access this essential, fundamental state of creative curiosity, I would suggest the judicious application of the archetypal energies of tenderness, fierceness and humour. To master this, practise on yourself. 20 minutes, twice a day. Give yourself your best attention, become aware of yourself, subtly, non-judgmentally, with creative curiosity, allow your present state to come into awareness, and go with the flow.

Your state

Summing up

Your state is the sum total of your neurological and biological processing at any one instant, and is key to the outcome of your consulting. Accessing resourceful states can be practised and mastered. Creating a supportive environment in the consultation, initially of non-judgmental acceptance of the content, and then developing and maintaining a state of creative curiosity in yourself at the outset, gives you the best chance of catalysing a fruitful consultation.

References

Covey S. (1989) *The Seven Habits of Highly Effective People* Free Press, New York, USA

ISBN 0-7432-6951-9

Balint M. (1964) *The Doctor, His Patient and The Illness* 2nd Edition Churchill Livingstone, London, UK ISBN 9780443064609

Gilligan S. (2002) *The Legacy of Milton H.Erickson* Selected papers of 2002 Zeig, Tucker and Theisen Inc, Phoenix, AZ 85016 ISBN 978-1-891944-90-1

Epicetus (1916) *The Enchiridion of Epicetus* (translated Matheson PE) Enhanced Media ISBN 978-1503226944

Frankl V. (1959) *Man's Search for Meaning* Rider Books, London, UK ISBN 978-1846043062

Grinder J. (2001) *Whispering in the Wind* J and C Enterprises ISBN 978-0971722309

Hanh T. (2008) *The Miracle of Mindfulness* Rider Books, London, UK ISBN 978-1-84-604106-8

Csikszentmihalyi M. (1992) *Flow* Random House, 20 Vauxhall Bridge Road London SW1V 2SA ISBN 9780712657594

A bedside manner

CHAPTER 2 - Rapport

"Disease occurs when the conscious and unconscious minds are out of rapport."
Milton Erickson

"Until we make the unconscious conscious it will control our destiny and we will call it fate."
Carl Jung

I had a registrar once who was struggling with time-keeping. We decided to look at this in a tutorial. We watched a video of some of her consultations to see if we could spot some areas to work on. She quickly noticed that she was doing most of the talking in the consultations, amongst other things we discussed the use of silence on the part of the doctor as a means of drawing out the patient, especially early in the consultation. I was supervising her evening surgery the same day. I noticed that a particular patient had been added as an extra at the end of her surgery. I was aware that this patient had a history of major depression and was curious as to how this would go. I was half-expecting to be asked to help at some point.

This didn't happen. At the end of surgery my registrar came to see me for the usual review session and she was in a state of some excitement. She told me she had just had "the best" consultation. The patient had come into her room. She had indicated the patient's chair in silence, as we had discussed. He sat down and said nothing. She resisted the temptation to say anything. After a while the patient relaxed back into the chair, with a pensive expression and they both maintained silence. After about 10 minutes of this, the patient suddenly smiled, stood up, said: "Thank you Doctor" and breezed happily out of the room.

So, what was going on here? I'll tell you in this chapter. First, we need to understand the concept of rapport. The term rapport stems from a French word meaning "to bring back". For an individual this means a harmonious internal connection between thought, feeling and action. In the context of interacting with patients, this means an energetic connection between the clinician and the patient extending beyond verbal interaction. It's what we mean when we say we are "on the same page" as someone. To take this a little further: Chambers 21st Century Dictionary (where else would I look?) defines rapport as: "a feeling of sympathy and understanding. A close emotional bond." I think this is a good starting point. It acknowledges the Primacy of Affect. Our first access is emotional and felt in the body.

In the last chapter, I discussed the importance of accessing the most resourceful state in oneself to prepare for meeting with the patient. This can be framed as the first step in establishing rapport with oneself. This implies setting a congruent and pure intention in oneself, and having all parts of the self, conscious and unconscious, aimed at delivering this. My preferred definition of rapport is the state that exists when the conscious and unconscious minds of all concerned are connected and in harmony. This allows for the concept of being in rapport with oneself, which is itself a pre-requisite for establishing rapport with anyone else.

Rapport

Putting theory into practice

In any encounter, in any context, there are two factors that are key to determining the quality of the outcome. These are the quality of the relationship between the participants, and their motivation. In the medical consultation this latter factor frequently amounts to the patient's willingness to engage and be pro-active in his or her own care. (I will discuss motivation in a later chapter). Now we are going to look at how the doctor can optimise the level of engagement of all parties involved in the consultation and best enhance the consultation's effectiveness. The root of this is rapport. Establishing rapport early in any interaction is key to obtaining a successful outcome for all parties.

From rapport flows trust, credibility, confidence and influence. In simple terms I am suggesting that rapport can be equated with "liking". In any exchange where the aim is change, the first step to helping people towards desired change is that they must like you. People buy the salesperson before they buy the product. People like people like them. If people like you, they will feel good around you and are far more likely to respond positively to the suggestions that arise in the exchange. As Robert B. Cialdini (Cialdini, 2001) has identified, liking is a key factor in influence. It is also increasingly recognised that people tend to make decisions emotionally and based around their values, rather than through any logical, deductive process. Once your own state is right, having people like you is the next step to helping them evolve, choose options, and, crucially, take appropriate action.

Having accessed your own best state of creative curiosity the next step then is to check that you are attuned to yourself; that your mind and body are in harmony. Having set the intention to use the time you have with your patient to help them to the best of your ability, it is vital to make sure that your own integrity is protected in the process. To do this a process of grounding and centering the self in the present moment, while establishing a shield around your own personality, so no harm of a physical, psychological, emotional or spiritual nature can come to you in your professional interactions is necessary. Once this self-attunement is in place, your full attention can be given to the situation in hand.

Remember that states are contagious. Once you have established this state in yourself this will be communicated in many ways, mostly unconscious, to your patient. The better the level of rapport you have established with them, the more efficient the process.

We are all aware of those consultations where, although we have done everything correctly by the book, things have not gone smoothly or just do not seem to have gone well for no apparent reason. The explanation for this is often that the appropriate level of rapport has not been achieved. So, let's look at how we get good rapport.

Establishing rapport

The first few seconds of any meeting are key to this. The warmth generated in this time leads to trust and respect, which themselves lead to confidence in your competence to help. If this opportunity is missed, it is very difficult, if not impossible to recover the ground subsequently. The most important skill in this context, and throughout all encounters, professional and otherwise, is precise calibration. This includes: watching, listening and tuning in to every bit of information that is being sent your way. The vast majority of this exchange is unconscious, hence the need for the shielding described above.

Rapport

As previously stated, the single most important gift you can give repeatedly is the quality of your attention, and this is particularly important in these first few seconds. Accurate observation and interpretation (calibration) of the patient's posture and movement is paramount. Specifically, we are concerned with: breathing rate and pattern, gestures, facial expressions, eye movements, and listening to the modulation of the patient's voice (pitch, tone, pace and volume).

These things give a huge and essential amount of information. Reflecting these back in your own physiology and communication is the key to building rapport, and when appropriate, communicating empathy. Now you've got that, let's break it down and look at the individual components of building rapport.

Words

Look and listen to the words the patient uses. These will give you many clues to how they are constructing their experience. Listen for their predicates: the words that tell you which senses they are using to decipher their experience. Here are some examples:
- "I feel ill . . ."
- "No one "listens" to me . . ."
- "I cannot see a way forward . . ."

Remember that people like people like them. If you then respond in their "language" your message will get through far more readily than if you do not. (Indeed, deliberately using a sensory modality that they are not is a good way of breaking rapport, if and when this is required.) Some rapport-building responses to the above examples might be:
- "How do you feel about this idea?"
- "I hear what you are saying, how does this idea sound?"

○ "How does this idea look to you?

This is a very dynamic situation. People change their preferred representational system constantly. Once you are tuned into this you can vary your responses accordingly and significantly help the conversation to flow. The common representational systems are illustrated in the examples I have used just now: visual, auditory and "kinaesthetic" (touch, feeling and movement). Others are taste and smell.

Linguistic calibration can be taken much further than this. Patients will communicate a lot of information about the values and beliefs they use to form their perception of their world by how they express themselves. Effective work involves identifying these values and beliefs and working with them, or helping the patient to update the ones which are no longer helping them, thus developing different frames for them to build on. The necessary sensibility and flexibility comes with practice. The first step is awareness that this abundant information is there to be identified and used.

We are meaning-making machines

From these observations a model can be constructed of how the patient is perceiving and interpreting their experience. From this understanding emerges a template on which you can build your responses. Everyone has their own unique way of perceiving the world: their own unique filters. These filters include their preferred representational system in any given context at any specific time, their values, beliefs, biases and preferred methods of choosing responses, and their intentions and motives.

Human beings are meaning-making machines. Stuff happens and we like to "make sense of it": to make a subjective interpretation.

Rapport

Transderivational search is a term used in psychology to describe the process of attaching meaning and hence words to experience by processing our perceptions through our memory bank and making associations with what is already there. The evidence of this process is there in the ways people express their understanding of the world, both to themselves (internal dialogue) and explicitly by language, both linguistic and physiological.

The conscious mind can process only about seven pieces of sensory information at any instant (Miller, 1956). There is an infinite amount of information available to us in every waking moment. What we choose to pay attention to is key to our experience and the outcomes we achieve. The information we focus on, and how we "make sense" of it, our "map", determines how we feel, and consequently, respond and act. Alfred Korzybski, the creator of the field of General Semantics, described reality as an "abstraction". (Korzybski, 1933)

It is important to understand that people's representation is not the whole reality. One way of putting this is the phrase: "the map is not the territory". For a map or model to be accurate in every detail it would have to be life-size. To make our maps and models, to make sense of our experience, essentially, we use three devices:

1. **Deletion**: leaving stuff out. As discussed above, at any one time we can only process a very limited amount of information. A process of selection of all the sensory input available to us occurs in our unconscious mind. An analogy would be shining a powerful torch into the night. Only what is within the torch's beam will be illuminated. The vast majority of what is out there will not. By moving the beam, new information becomes available as some disappears from view. Our experience is entirely dependent on where we place our attention: where we

point the torch.

2. **Distortion**: distorted information is ambiguous and often abstract. Assumptions and judgements are presented without the supporting corroborative information. Examples could be: "He did not buy me flowers. He does not love me." This is called a complex-equivalence and we can ask: "How does not buying flowers equate to not loving some one?" Another example could be: "I have acne, so no one will ask me out." Here we see cause and effect and we can ask if the cause is really leading to that effect. Listening particularly for cause-effect and complex-equivalence relationships is a quick way of identifying the beliefs and values that motivate people and drive their experience. The effective patterns can then be reinforced and the limiting patterns gently challenged to allow alternatives to emerge. This process is called reframing.

3. **People also generalise**. Generalisation is where patterns and consistency are assumed. An example might be a universal quantifier such as: "Nobody likes me".

Patterns and perception

Once these patterns are identified it is possible to build rapport by acknowledging them, summarising them, and thus pacing the patient's experience. This information can also be used to challenge some of the identified patterns and help them become aware that there are different ways of perceiving their experience. Paraphrasing Rudyard Kipling:

> *I have seven helpful little friends,*
> *I use them now and then.*
> *They are: How? and Which? and What and Who?*
> *And Why? and Where? and When? (Kipling, 1902)*

That takes us on to questions and how we ask them.

Rapport

Asking better questions

A way to further establish rapport is to ask good questions. Once an appreciation of how people may be forming their experience of their world has been attained, appropriate questions can be formulated. This will enable you to tease out more details of how they are making their map/model and help them identify ways this may be modified to be more useful now. Let's look at how we can do this. Deletions can be questioned. To clarify a deletion, ask for the missing information. Here is an example, the patient says: "They say we should all be eating . . ." Perhaps you can ask: "Who says?" (Who specifically? What specifically?)

Distortions can be questioned by seeking clarification, by asking: "How specifically?" Here are some examples, the patient says, "He makes me so cross," you can ask "How does he do this?" With a generalisation, look for the exception. If the patient says, "I am tired all the time," probe this, ask "All the time?" or if the patient says, "No-one likes me," question them, "No-one?"

Body-language

Even more important than calibrating people's words is to tune into what their physiology is saying. The body keeps the score. Our first response to our experience is affective. We feel before we think. Autonomic and affective reactions, with their somato-sensory manifestations, occur significantly before any cognitive processing occurs. Our conscious mind becomes engaged at a definite interval after our unconscious has responded to whatever is happening.

This has obvious survival value. We are much indebted to the work of Dr Hans Selye in the 1930s in Montreal (Viner, 1999). Cortisol had been identified as a hormone produced as part of his General Adaptation Syndrome in response to what he described as "stress" (another metaphor borrowed from engineering science: the application of a force to a material). He described the "flight, fight and fright" response that is mediated by a surge in cortisol production from the adrenal glands, and that characterises our unconscious and immediate response to a threat. The physical signs of dilated pupils, pallor and increased respiratory rate are all visible evidence that this process is taking place. The racing heart can be picked up in the pulse rate and is often described by the patient.

What eye movements can tell you

It has long been observed that people's eyes move unconsciously in different directions, according to what they are thinking. This is an area where calibration is again key, as this is unique to each individual, and, even then, not necessarily consistent from context to context.

Typically, if the instantaneous and spontaneous eye-movement is up, often the patient is processing information visually. Side-to-side movement suggests they are processing using auditory systems. Characteristically, eye-movement to the left indicates that attention is in the past: they are "remembering". Eye movement to the right suggest future-focus, constructing. In some people the past is to their right and the future to their left, so if you are exploring this, remember to calibrate and check from time to time.

Looking down to the right suggests kinaesthetic processing "feeling". (I suspect this is where the saying "down-right", as in "down-right miserable" in idiomatic English usage comes from.) Looking down and to the left (the "telephone position") implies that internal dialogue is taking place. The patient is having a discussion with themselves in their head. It is generally a good idea to respect this and not interrupt, or perhaps to ask "What are you thinking?" after an interval. Very often they will respond without questioning how you knew they were thinking anything at all!

Matching, Pacing and Leading

All the information gleaned by calibrating your patient thus can then be used to match their language, both spoken and body, subtly. Matching their physiology is possibly even more important than using their preferred verbal representational system. Adopting a similar posture and mirroring their micro-movements and, particularly, matching their respiratory rate and using consistent predicates and representational systems in your language are all very effective ways of communicating to their unconscious mind that you are on their wave-length.

People like people like them. This is sometimes called pacing their experience. You can test how effectively you are doing this by subtly changing something, such as a slight shift in posture, and seeing if they, unconsciously do the same. This is described as leading. This has to be done very careful and subtly. If it is done too overtly they will become consciously aware of it, rapport will be broken and a lot of ground will need to be made up.

There is a variant of matching which is even more subtle. This is known as cross-mirroring. While mirroring describes doing the same movements as the patient, including matching their respiratory rate, cross-mirroring means picking up on something they are doing and doing something yourself. This needs to remain consistent. Whenever they do "A", you do "B". This is particularly useful when the behaviour they are doing is undesired. For example, if your patient is very agitated or distressed, their breathing and movements may be very disordered. Instead of trying to match their breathing rate you can pace it with another movement such as a nod of the head with each expiration, or pacing with your finger, like a subtle orchestra conductor. Once rapport is established you can modulate the pace of your movements and thus help the patient find a more resourceful state as their behaviour responds to your lead. This is a good test of rapport. Matching needs to be done subtly, but it is worth the practice and effort. As Heraclitus said long ago: "An unapparent communication is stronger than an apparent one." This is still true today.

Summing up

Establishing rapport both with yourself and with your patient is essential to any successful outcome. Milton Erickson framed the job of the doctor as creating the environment (the weather) wherein the patient can reconnect their conscious and unconscious minds: disease (dis-ease) being the manifestation of these being out of rapport, and the indication that something needs to be done to reconnect them.

We have looked at how rapport can be achieved by accurate calibration of the information a patient is constantly giving us, both verbally and non-verbally, consciously and most importantly, unconsciously. Voltaire said: "men use words to disguise their thoughts." Being alert and aware to the unconscious cues we are being sent is essential.

Rapport

This information helps us to build rapport by matching and pacing our patients, and ultimately guiding them forward, elegantly, efficiently and effectively.

A note of caution

Rapport is not the same as empathy or compassion, although there is sometimes confusion around the usage of these terms.
I understand compassion to mean a mutual capacity for anguish and suffering: literally "suffering with". Sympathy means "suffering like", parallel processing if you like. Empathy means literally "the same suffering".

I referred earlier in this chapter to the importance of shielding the ego from potential harm from _____ cesses occurring in the consultation. It is perhaps in th_____ _____thy that this is most important. We can walk in st_____ _____on their journey, but we cannot do it for th_____ _____ children by doing their homework f_____ _____fe place within ourselves to b_____ _____ so our unconscious wisdo_____ _____ cify how best to process w_____ _____ given back. Empathy is im_____ _____ed and used judiciously. _____ _____y, and a very important_____ _____ yourself, is the equally-_____ _____u do seriously, with great _____

This raises _____ _____nother term borrowed from engineering. T_____ _____naterial to stress. Too much empathy, injudicio_____ _____s a very quick root to exhaustion, burnout, helplessness _____ disillusionment. The antidote to empathy is often laughter. Limbic resonance is a term used to describe the situation when the conscious and unconscious mind are in rapport. The outward manifestation of this is the smile.

In Conclusion

I opened this chapter with a story about an apparently successful consultation conducted in silence by my registrar and her patient. During our tutorial that same day we had discussed building rapport using verbal and particularly non-verbal cues from the patient and how much harder it is to detect and calibrate these when we are doing the talking; focusing on what we want to say rather than the information the patient is giving us, verbal and non-verbal. My registrar was a very quick learner and took the opportunity to find for herself just how effective it can be just to observe, calibrate, match and pace. No leading was required in that situation. The doctor provided the environment for the patient to do the work they needed on that occasion. The day ended with smiles all round.

Further Reading

The first useful insights I gained in studying and building rapport came when I was training to be a GP Trainer in 1993. One of the books we were encouraged to read was:

The Inner Consultation by Dr Roger Neighbour
There is now a 2nd Edition
2005 Radcliffe Publishing Ltd
ISBN: 1-85775 679 7

I have re-read this book many times over the years since I first found it. A real game-changer for me. The book makes many references to the work of Richard Bandler and John Grinder, whose collaborative work in the 1970s became Neuro-Linguistic Programming (NLP).

Much of the detail in this chapter comes from what I have learned through studying and training in NLP. There are innumerable sources of information available about NLP. The two co-founders are still training people 40 years later. If this floats your boat I would suggest starting with them and Roger Neighbour's book.

Among the earliest publications were:

The Structure of Magic by Richard Bandler and John Grinder
1975 Science and Behaviour Books, Inc
ISBN: 08314-0044-7

The Structure of Magic II by Richard Bandler and John Grinder
1976 Science and Behaviour Books, Inc
ISBN: 08314-0049-8

Frogs into Princes by Richard Bandler and John Grinder
1979 Real People Press
ISBN: 0-911226-19-2

References

Cialdini R. (2001) *Influence: Science and Practice*
4th Edition Allyn and Bacon ISBN 0-321-01147-3

Miller G. (1956*) The Magical Number Seven, Plus or Minus Two. Some limits on our capacity for processing information*. (Princeton University Department of Psychology) Psychological Review 63 (2): 81-97.

Korzybski A. (1933) *Science and Sanity: An Introduction to Non-Aristotelian Systems and General Semantics* First published in 1933 5th Edition 1994 Institute of General Semantics ISBN 0-685-406161-4

A bedside manner

Viner R. (1999) *Putting Stress in Life: Hans Selye and the Making of Stress Theory: Social Studies of Science.* 29 (3): 391-410

Kipling R. (1902) *I Keep Six Honest Serving Men, Just So Stories : The Elephant's Child* Wordsworth Editions Ltd. ISBN 10: 1 85326 102 5

CHAPTER 3 - Their State

This chapter explores the importance of the patient's state in establishing an effective working relationship and helping them achieve results. Here, I discuss what the doctor can do to ensure the patient can access the most useful states in themselves to generate successful outcomes to the consultation process.

In Chapter 1, I argued that the single most important factor in achieving an outcome is our state. This applies to the patient just as much as to the doctor. There are so many anecdotal accounts of times when people are able to achieve apparently super-human results. A mother lifting a car to free her child from underneath it; a French man who ate an aeroplane. Innumerable tales of apparent miracles of endurance and survival. The key to all these is the ability to generate resourceful states at the appropriate times. In Chapter 1, I explored in detail how important your state is in optimising your ability to help yourself and, in the professional context, help others. I also raised the issue of parallel processing. States are contagious. It is thus important to be flexible and to be able to access and adapt resourceful states in yourself, as you will pass these on to your patient. It is equally important to build safety and protection into your state so that you are protected from unhelpful and dangerous state transference from your patient.

Much of what I said in that chapter is also relevant to helping your patient access their most appropriate states to best facilitate their learning, growth, adaptation and change. Our experience of life, and thus our state, (the sum total of our thoughts and feelings at any given moment), are entirely a function of where we place our focus.

When helping new registrars approach how to build an effective, efficient and elegant consultation style, I refer back to Stephen Covey's (Covey, 1989) advice: start with the end in mind. How do you want the patient to feel at the end of the consultation? What do you want them to be saying? I am reminded of the episode with the Cheshire Cat in *Alice's Adventures in Wonderland*, where Alice, at a junction, asks which road to take. The Cat asks her where she wants to go. Alice says she does not know, to which the Cat replies that in that case it doesn't matter which way she goes. (Lewis Caroll, 1865)

I have already talked about how failing to build good rapport is a stumbling block in consulting successfully. Another stumbling block is failing to set good objectives. This will be covered in a lot more detail in a subsequent chapter. Suffice to say here that the first objective is for the patient to get their state right.

I often suggest to the registrars that, as a starting point for the consultation, to have in mind what you want the patient to be saying at the end of the consultation. Something along the lines of: "I feel better just for talking to you."? That seems a reasonable and realistic objective for a ten-minute interaction. This brings us back, yet again, to the Primacy of Affect. To paraphrase Maya Angelou: long after people have forgotten what you said and did, they will remember how you made them feel.

Their state

This is pre-cognitive. In my view an important part of a doctor's job is to help people get better (note the deletion: what specifically does 'better' mean? Better than what? How specifically will they know they are better?). I believe having the patient 'spontaneously' express a sentiment along these lines is a good aim for the doctor to have at the outset of a consultation. This is a reflection of a good, resourceful state in the patient, itself a product of the gentle, compassionate and caring attitude of the doctor performing optimally. Bearing in mind my thoughts on parallel processing, as I frame the consultation as a learning experience, the same state of creative curiosity as I recommend for the doctor is also appropriate for the patient, and will communicate itself. What is their unconscious trying to communicate? How can we best meet it and learn from it? I have found Stephen Gilligan's teaching in this area particularly helpful. My understanding of this is that the patient often presents to us in a **CRASH** state.

Constricted: their focus is narrowed and dominated by their 'problem'. Their focus is often very much in the present, with little, if any awareness of where things are likely to lead if left unchecked. The initial work is often to 'dehypnotise' them and help them out of their 'illness-trance'.

Reactive: They are often responding moment-to-moment in their lives, unaware of the bigger picture. They are so busy counting the beans that they are forgetting to taste the stew. They are task-oriented rather than strategy-oriented.

Analysing: Paralysis by analysis. Stuck in their cognitive, analytic assessment of their situation, they have no access to their own creativity.

Separated: from their resources. Hippocrates said that it is natural resources within us which are the true healers of disease.

It is our job to help our patients restore contact with their own inner wisdom, and all the resources, internal and external, that are available to them.

Hurt and hurting: States are contagious. The suffering and anguish our patients are experiencing are not usually confined just to themselves, but spread out into those they are in contact with. Helping the patient helps many others simultaneously.

I have already referred to the shielding necessary to protect ourselves from 'catching' any of this from our patients. One of the effective ways to do this is to access the appropriate resolution state ourselves, the **COACH** state and pass this on to our patient

Centered: our strength and thinking rooted in our own best resources and grounded and shielded from harm. **Open**: receptive to all the information available to us. This enables the necessary, precise calibration available in an optimised state of clarity and positive intention. This permits unconditional positive regard, that is only possible in the context of firm boundaries, rules of engagement and pure intention. **Aware**: an optimised state of paying attention. Subtle, non-judgmental awareness spread uniformly and globally. Being aware of the patient, of ourselves, and of the infinite reservoir of resources available to us: internally and externally, temporally and historically. This is the basis of the Mindfulness identified by Thich Nhat Hanh (Hanh, 2008) and which is the basis of a considerable array of contemporary interventions. **Connected**: connected to all the resources discussed above. **Holding**: capable of creating and maintaining a space between doctor and patient where new outcomes can arise, germinate, grow and develop.

Sponsorship

The work here could be described as helping people move from survival mode to mindful mode.

There are echoes here of the work of Selye (Selye, 1956), the Hungarian-Canadian endocrinologist and his work with cortisol in Montreal in the mid-1930s. Cortisol had only recently been isolated and identified. He coined the term 'stress' (another metaphor from engineering), and described the "Orienting" Response, the state of flight, fright and fight: the amygdala-based response to threat. This is pre-cognitive and instinctual and, in most animals, this can only be sustained briefly. The fright produces an appropriate response, fight or flight, and relaxation is then possible. The only animal who can sustain the Orienting Response indefinitely appears to be homo-sapiens.

We are now well aware of the harmful effects on many aspects of our health of these prolonged, raised cortisol levels and the associated endocrine and physiological responses. This Orienting Response corresponds in many ways to the CRASH state described above.

The reciprocal and desirable COACH state can be learned, practised and mastered by regular assiduous practice and I would suggest that it is a hallmark of any effective intervention that the patient develops this habit of optimising their coping state by some form of regular practice. This is a skill, and like any skill, can be improved and augmented by learning and practice. To this optimised COACH state can be added several other useful states, including safety, nurturing, wisdom, self-esteem, confidence and optimism, as well as the essential archetypal energies of tenderness, fierceness and playfulness. There is more on this later in the book.

If this is achieved, it brings resilience: the ability to withstand stress. Victor Frankl (Frankl, 1959) identified an important aspect of this, particularly in the context of suffering, as the ability to give meaning to experience. The cognitive aspect of this work is best done in an optimised learning state. When we are aware of unresourceful states in ourselves and others there are a few things we can usefully do to improve the situation. As always, our results are a result of where we place our focus.

A useful starting point is physiology. States usually last for about 90 seconds unless we do something to reinforce them. We often maintain state with our posture and facial expression. For example, smiling or whistling when happy, and frowning when unhappy or deep in thought. 'The body keeps the score,' is a Buddhist idea so fundamental to the art of the practice of medicine. Fortunately, the system works in reverse too. We can alter our state immediately by altering our physiology. Try putting on a smile and feeling sad. We could try to help our patients by making direct suggestions about postural changes. This, however, is not guaranteed, or even likely, to be met with much success.

There is a better way, if we have established and maintained rapport we can achieve results by modulating our own posture. Our patient's mirror neurones (Rizzolatti, Craighero, 2004) will pick this up and produce a matching response in their physiology. Information communicated indirectly is far more effective than information communicated directly, as Heraclitus told us many years ago, or, as Gandhi put it: "Be the change that you want to see in the world.".

Another avenue is to consider the verbal language used. Changing a single word in a sentence, or even just the inflections and emphasis, can profoundly change the interpretation and meaning the patient gives it. A simple example would be to substitute the word 'discomfort' for the word 'pain'; "As I examine your hand you may feel some pain," can become: "As I examine your hand you may feel some discomfort,". This needs to be done subtly and with good calibration of the patient's response. What is said has to be plausible.

A third way of helping people alter their state is by directing their focus. If the patient is undergoing a potentially uncomfortable procedure, having them focus elsewhere, perhaps on a happy memory or some keenly-anticipated event in the future is likely to distract them from the discomfort of the present and help their tolerance.

Summary

This chapter has looked at the importance of the patient's state and how to help this. When doctor and patient are both in optimised, resourced, learning states (creative curiosity) and in rapport with themselves and each other, good results can be anticipated.

References

Covey S. (1989) *The Seven Habits of Highly Effective People* Free Press, New York, USA

ISBN 0-7432-6951-9

Carroll L.. (1865) *Alice's Adventures in Wonderland* Collins Classics ISBN 1908760748

Hanh T. (2008) *The Miracle of Mindfulness* Rider Books, London, UK

ISBN 978-1-84-604106-8

Selye H. (1956) *The Stress of Life* McGraw-Hill Education ISBN 9780070562127

Frankl V. (1959) *Man's Search for Meaning* Rider Books, London, UK ISBN 184413239

Rizzolatti G.; Craighero L. (2004) *Mirror Neurones*

http://www.kuleuven.be/mirrorneuronsystem/readinglist/Rizzolatti%20&%20Craighero
%202004%20-%20The%20MNS%20-%20ARN.pdf (PDF). *Annual Review of Neuroscience*.
27 (1): 169-192. https://doi.org/10.1146%2Fannurev.neuro.27.070203.144230 (accessed
15/04/2018)

CHAPTER 4 - Hope

In this chapter I will develop some ideas about hope: why it is important and how to help patients find it where possible.

Very early in my career I came across a quote attributed to the priest and author C.S. Lewis: "It is never too late to have a dream, never too late to make a plan." This made a profound impression on me and taught me the importance of instilling hope in our patients wherever possible. This does not mean that I am encouraging raising false hope or deliberately misleading patients with inaccurate or unrealistic predictions, but rather engaging with them in ways that allow them to reframe their experience into something potentially constructive or interesting, if not enjoyable, even if only in the very short-term. I have spent time at the bedside in the last day of a patient's life listening to them talking about their children and grand-children and what life may hold for them. Vicarious hope perhaps but generating good chemistry, some endorphin release in an otherwise-troubled brain. Even in the last days of a terminal illness people can find peace and comfort in the instant.

One of the most important duties of the doctor is to inspire and reinforce hope in the patient. This is a delicate and skilful task, which requires diligence, honesty and integrity. While it is inappropriate to inspire false hope, it is almost always possible to help patients identify perspectives and frames they had not considered, and help them identify potential positives for themselves or others, in most situations. In this way we can help them access resources, personal and external, that they were previously unaware they had available to them. In this respect it is important to be aware that there is always the possibility of some sort of positive outcome in all but the most dire of situations. Some patients develop a certain 'gallows humour' and can find aspects of their situation to laugh about, often in the most difficult situations. I do not discourage this. On the contrary, it is a way they have found to ease their burden and, where appropriate, I will laugh with them.

Whatever problem is being faced, somewhere in there will be the seeds of a solution. It is far easier to re-direct a stream than to dam it up, so the trick is to be curious and explore whatever the patient brings, as this will contain the information that will lead to the generation of the solution. This is the principle of utilisation.

Viktor Frankl identified the natural human attribute of seeking to give meaning to our experience. This is not primarily a logical process and requires the use of the imagination too. When we are able to give meaning to our suffering we are able to build resilience and find the resources we need to cope and learn and heal. In Buddha's words: "Pain is inevitable. Suffering is optional." What turns pain in to suffering is resistance. If we can help people to learn to accept the aspects of their situation that they cannot change, this allows them to direct their focus, intention and energies on optimising their experience of what lies ahead. If resistance is replaced with creative curiosity, then learning, growth and change can happen. There is no substitute for giving the patient the time and opportunity, when they are ready, to explore their experiences and reflections on them, and match them up with their values. This allows them the opportunity to review their values and perhaps do a bit of updating, so they can bring some positivity to the next stage.

Sir William Osler, a Canadian physician of a century ago charged us that it is the duty of the doctor to: "cure sometimes, alleviate often, and to comfort always". We must always be aware of the effect that our words and communication are having on our patients, and take every care to communicate in a kind, sensitive, compassionate and considerate way. This starts with, and is impossible without, listening thoroughly to them at the outset, and gaining rapport. From listening comes understanding and compassion and from compassion flows healing, which often involves forgiveness, of ourselves and others.

We must always be on the look-out for opportunities to build and sustain hope in our patients, and avoid anything, however well-intentioned, which dashes it. This is particularly relevant in the context of General Practice. In the UK National Health Service, the patient remains always under the care of their GP. When the secondary services (hospital and specialist care) are involved, the patient's contact with the GP can be minimal. There often comes a point where the patient has completed the lines of therapy and intervention appropriate to their condition, but the underlying issues are not resolved. Along the way there may or may not have been significant involvement with the GP, but there frequently comes a point where the conventional, evidence-based medical armoury has been exhausted, but there is still much to be done. This is not to suggest that an evidence-based approach be abandoned, but the patient needs much more than this. In the introduction in this book, I referred to the art of medicine and it is in this context that this becomes highly relevant. Sir William Osler also observed that one of the factors that distinguishes humans from the rest of the animal kingdom is their desire to take medication. There is much more to medicine than the provision of medication. Medicine is not something you give, it is something you do: a practice and a set of skills. An art. Palliative and end-of-life care are contexts where the GP's role can have a profound impact on the patient's experience.

Asymptotic medicine

An opportunity for some constructive direction of focus and reframing occurs when a patient with cancer has had a difficult consultation about their prognosis. Five-year survival is the conventional way of looking at the situation and the patient advised of the percentage chance of being alive five years from the diagnosis. This will be influenced by the stage of the disease. As people succumb the line on the graph moves down towards the base line. Unless five-year survival is zero, the line does not meet the base line and never will. The area between the base line and the graph is the asymptote. If patients are aware of this, rather than dwell on where the statistics place them in terms of five-year survival, I suggest they focus their attention on the people in the asymptote and see if they can work out how to be one of these people. A gentle reframe that has them focused on survival and offers them some hope.

Summary

This chapter has illustrated the importance of instilling hope, where possible, into the consulting process. Once all parties are in good states, rapport is established and there is hope, we are a long way to generating a fruitful consultatio

CHAPTER 5 - Goal-Setting

"Start with the end in mind." Stephen Covey

The importance of having some direction in the consultation has already been identified in previous chapters. In this chapter, I will discuss the nature of the goals we are talking about and give some pointers about setting them congruently.

When reflecting on consultations that have not gone well, I find that a fairly consistent feature has been that no clear mutual goal-setting has gone on. A goal in this context is a desired outcome. What are we trying to achieve? Patients often present in a state of distress. Their attention is often focused on their experience of misery and suffering. If they are focused on what has happened this often produces low mood and 'depression'.

If they are anticipating the future consequences of their problems, this often contributes to anxiety. We do them a great service when we do something as simple as shift their focus from their problem state to their desired outcomes. The Miracle Question (De Shazer, 1988) is a very helpful short cut here. Simply stated this can be paraphrased as: "How will you be when you no longer have the problem?" To answer this, the patient has to leave the problem frame and use their imagination to create a desired future. In Chapter 3, while discussing the patient's state, I mentioned the idea of starting with the end in mind: what we want the patient to be feeling at the end of the consultation. If we set goals for ourselves in our consulting and achieve rapport with our patients as we do it, they will start doing the same thing.

The traditional teaching in coaching uses the S.M.A.R.T (Doran, 1981) model for goal-setting. This was a model developed by George Doran, a business management consultant, to help companies prepare management goals and objectives. His original criteria were that these goals should be specific, measurable, assignable, realistic and time-framed. This model has stood the test of time in business practice and has been used as the basis for many subsequent models in life-coaching practice. However, in my view, the absence of an ecology check limits its value for use when setting congruent goals for individuals or groups.

I prefer to use a different mnemonic for setting congruent goals for myself and my patients: D.E.P.O.S.E.R.S

- Direction
- Ecology
- Positive
- Own resources
- Specific
- Evidence-based
- Resourced
- Size

Let us look at these criteria in some more detail.

Direction
Direction is the first on the list for a good reason. The most important aspect of having a goal is that it gives us direction. This gets us proactive. We have something, somewhere to be aiming

for in the present moment. When we have a direction to go in, we can set off purposefully. One of the beauties of this goal-setting process is that we do not have to achieve the goals we set. The job of these goals is to get us proactive and doing something constructive. That is enough. It is often the case that, as we near a goal, it loses its appeal, as something even more compelling comes into sight. This is OK. This goal-setting process is continuous, requiring regular reflection and re-calibration, hour-by-hour, day-by-day. Very often patients are patients because of where they are aiming themselves. Some gentle, judicious assistance in nudging the rudder from time to time can pay huge dividends.

Ecology

Whatever goals we choose need to be ecologically sound. That is, they preserve and develop the current resources and beneficial aspects of our lives, and even build on them. Goal-setting may be going on in several different aspects of our lives at the same time. It is important that we maintain an awareness of any potential conflicts. A goal may satisfy all the other criteria, but if it is not ecologically sound it is not going to be congruent (the right thing, at the right time, in the right place, for the right people).

Positive

State goals in the positive. It is not possible to achieve a negative goal. Ask: "What do you want?" Not: "What do you not want?" When we start to discuss goal-setting with a patient they will often reply with an 'away-from' answer. "I don't want . . .". This helps in that it gives us information to help build rapport: their preferred way of presenting their wishes at that point is in terms of 'away-from'. This is OK to a point. It brings us to where Alice was in Chapter 3. 'Away-from' requires less emotional energy than 'towards' and is an essential part of the stress-response of flight, fright and fight. It has survival value, but is not constructive.

59

It provides a starting point. Developing an outcome-focus, stated in the positive early in the consultation, is important in using the time available efficiently.

Own resources

Any goal that relies on external resources is going to be highly dependent on the availability of these resources and hence vulnerable. Any goal that relies on other people's behaviour is doomed to failure. "I will be OK when my partner stops . . ." is never going to work long-term, and possibly not even in the short-term. An awareness of this criterion brings into play the importance of the patient taking responsibility for the outcomes they generate and being accountable to themselves for them. The more the patient commits to generating the desired outcome, the more likely they are to achieve it. Seek to generate sentences from them which start with: "I am going to have/be/do . . ." While the support of others undoubtedly helps individuals reach desired goals, success is ultimately in their own hands.

Specific

The more specific the definition of the goal is, the easier it is to plan what needs to be done to achieve it, and to measure progress. "I am going to start going to the gym more often," becomes much more likely to happen if it is stated as: "I am going to go to Gym X at 5.30 pm every Monday, Wednesday and Friday and do exercises A, B and C for 20 minutes each."

Evidence-based

This is not quite as obvious as it might appear. There are two aspects to this. The more obvious one is the external evidence that will show a goal has been achieved: what the individual and others will be able to observe if they look. For someone wishing to lose some weight this might be weighing 12 stone by Christmas or fitting comfortably into a Size 12 dress. Very good so far. At a subtler level, it helps greatly to attach emotions to goals. How will the person feel when they have achieved their goal: perhaps ask what 'gut reaction' will they be looking for when they have got there. Remember, the body keeps the score. They might get to the gym as illustrated above, but their body will tell them if they are working at it in the way that they should through their feelings and emotions. If the gym session is followed by a stop at a fast-food outlet or the pub on the way home, their feeling and emotions will not give them the thumbs-up they need. There will be more about this in the chapter on motivation later in the book.

Resourced

I have already touched on the importance of being self-reliant with regard to resources. One of the major challenges in achieving any goal is the allocation of time. Making appointments with the self for important activities is essential and helps reduce procrastination. Once external resources have been identified and mobilised, things such as gym membership, – help with school collection and child-minding – attention can be given to resourcing internally. We are back to where we started here, with accessing the right state and attitude set to deliver the results we want. The 'R' here could also stand for 'Realistic' and 'Relevant'. The individual's own self-calibration skill set are an essential resource, to check that they are staying on-track, and, if necessary, to bring themselves back on-track, or review their goals after due reflection.

Size

Goals need to be the right size. Too small and they are not motivating enough, too big and they become impossible or overwhelming. I suggest the optimum size is slightly outrageous. We are not going for perfection here, or even for achieving the goals we set ourselves. If they are to give us a direction to be heading in, they need to be compelling and by making them big and ambitious they will look attractive and, as and when we get anywhere near them, our achievements will be considerable and excellent. Once a goal or goals have been identified that are congruent for patient and doctor then we are well on the way to success. Sometimes goals will emerge which tick all the boxes for the patient, but which do not sit well with the doctor. It is important to be aware of this and respond to it. Either the goals need revising or the patient will need to seek help elsewhere. Otherwise the doctor's incongruence will sabotage the process. This will probably be at the point of building up motivation: the subject of the next chapter.

Summary

The conscious mind is best employed in planning the future. Setting congruent goals early in the consultation process and calibrating progress are key skills that contribute to the generation of satisfactory outcomes for ourselves and our patients. We are not seeking perfection here. The only perfection possible is in the purity of our intentions. This applies to doctor and patient. Once these intentions are clearly established negotiation of mutually agreeable and congruent goals can happen, with the objective of seeking the best outcomes possible. In another word: excellence.

References

De Shazer S. (1988) *The Miracle Question*

www.netzwerk ost.at/publikationen/pdf/miraclequestion.pdf (accessed 14/04/2018)

Doran G. (1981) *Smart Goals*

Management Review Magazine, November 1981. 70(11) 35-36

CHAPTER 6 - Motivation

Once someone has accessed the most appropriate state for their situation, the other factors that determine the likelihood of achieving their desired outcome are their expectation and particularly their motivation. Motivation generates drive and determination. The result is action, and the development of good habits. In this chapter, I will explore some ideas about motivation and how to introduce them into consulting.

Ultimately, everything is done for a feeling. I want to consult well because it gives me a feeling of satisfaction to see a patient make some significant, constructive changes in their life and achieve things they had thought impossible. Throughout my career I have frequently been surprised when people have thanked me for my help and I cannot remember anything I specifically did which helped them, other than provide a space for them to reflect, explore and find their own way forward. Once people have identified goals that have value for them, they will find their way towards them and enjoy the process, at least some of the time. They will also find the drive and motivation to keep going in the tough times too.

State

From what has already been said about state and rapport, it is clear that if the doctor is highly motivated to generate a good consultation, and help their patient towards some worthwhile outcomes, this will transmit itself to the patient. Similarly, the patient will have had times in their lives when they have been successful at something. Also, they will have skills and abilities and other resources that will help them, but which they may not be aware of. Gently reminding patients of all this by some gentle questioning will help them access a useful state which can then be aimed into the future by identifying the desired outcomes.

The Miracle Question has already been discussed in the last chapter. "How will you be when you no longer have the problem?" is a very effective question for focusing the attention of all parties on desired outcomes and evoking resourceful states. Essentially, we can change how we feel by changing what we believe is going to happen in the future. Encouraging our patients to focus their attention on how they want to be, to adopt the physical posture that matches it, rehearsing the way they are going to be talking to themselves in this state when the problems they are facing have been successfully resolved, and feeling the desired feelings are all potent ways of motivating them to start doing what they need to do to deliver. Once they have done this future rehearsal, the blueprint is already in the system and they will find it much easier to start to work towards delivering this.

Language

The language people use will provide clues as to how best to help them get on with the work of moving towards the goals they seek. We have already discussed how, when distressed, people will often express their wishes in terms of what they do *not* want. "I do not want to feel like this," would be an example. Their formulation of their wish is that they want to get away from something. This is a common default position. This is because it takes less mental and emotional effort to move away from something undesirable than it does to move towards something preferable. This is important. It is the limbic system at work and has vital life-saving and preserving functions. If our unconscious early-warning systems sense danger they move us away from the danger before we have time to 'think'. Once we are relatively safe our higher mental functions kick in and we start to formulate a linguistic explanation for what just happened. This is the 'carrot-and-stick' phenomenon. In general people will choose to avoid the stick rather than go for the carrot. Our job is to help them make the carrot more compelling than the stick-dodging.

This awareness gives us some options to help them make progress. When they have identified a desired goal, a way of making it potentially more attractive is to describe it in their 'away-from' language. For example, a smoker who wants to give up may respond best when all the aspects of life that they won't have as a result are identified. They won't have to worry about the damage they are doing to their health, they won't have to feel so breathless when they exercise, they won't have to worry about the smell of smoke on their clothes and breath etc.

Values and beliefs

Values are abstract concepts that are important to us and are often related to our core beliefs. Beliefs are what we 'know' to be true: a feeling of certainty about a thought. When a belief is expressed, there is always going to be a related value underlining it. Beliefs can be empowering or limiting.

When stated congruently, "I am strong," "I can cope with this," reveal empowering beliefs. "I am weak," "I cannot cope," are limiting beliefs, and can be gently challenged with counter examples from the individual's experiences. Identifying the values and beliefs which are driving or holding back our patient gives us very useful information to help them build their motivation.

Values work at a level more profound than the material world. For example, money is not a value. The value related to money might be abundance, or security. When people set congruent goals, one of the factors that make them congruent is that they are consistent with the person's values. A powerful and efficient way of eliciting people's values is to ask them what is important to them, and what makes it important to them. The trick here is to be persistent and keep asking: "What does that give you?" until a nominalisation, a verb turned into a noun, emerges. Then find out how they feel about that. Everything we do is done for a feeling. When the feeling is good, it is likely that an important underlying value for them has been identified.

The conversation might go along the lines of:

Doc: "What is most important to you in your life?"

Patient: "My family?"

Doc: "What feeling does thinking about your family give you?"

Patient: "Warmth"

Doc: "Anything else?"

Patient: "Contentment"

Doc: "Anything else?"

Motivation

Patient: "Security"

In this illustration contentment and security are values that have emerged. An important aspect of this exchange is accurate calibration. As the words emerge there will be a lot of changes in the patient's manner and physiology. The doctor needs to be watching closely and looking for congruity. When the body-language matches the words then a useful value has been identified.

This is an exercise worth repeating over and over ("What else is important?") in a session as several values will emerge and often the person's most important motivating values are not among the first one or two to be identified. When you have a list of perhaps six or eight, ask the person to rearrange them in order of importance. It is likely that their key driving values in their life will be the first few on the list.

Exploring the 'away-from' pattern discussed above can also be a good way of eliciting important values. "What do you tend to avoid in life?". Break it down as before, then prioritise the list as before. Values generate emotion (Latin: *move out-of*). Everything is done for a feeling. As Ry Cooder, the Californian musician, once observed: "Every dollar is spent on feeling good,". When key values can be attached to goals, the chances of action, progress and success are vastly increased by the associated emotional charge.

Drivers of motivation

The forces that influence motivation significantly are need, confidence and competence. People will be compelled to go for things they believe to be important. Beliefs differ from values, and value and belief sets are unique to each individual. As we have already seen, values are things we know to be important. Beliefs are things we know to be 'true'. I use parentheses because everyone has their own truths. Leon Festinger, an American social psychologist, coined the term "cognitive dissonance" (Festinger, 1957), for the uncomfortable feeling we get when our thoughts or actions conflict with a value we hold. We cannot tolerate it for long. We have to either review the value and see if it needs updating, or alter our thoughts or behaviour to something more congruent. Cognitive dissonance is a powerful motivator. We need to feel comfortable.

Our likelihood of taking appropriate action is greatly increased if we have the competence to do so. In the previous chapter on goal-setting, one of the factors identified was resources. These may include education, training and practice. As competence grows, so will the confidence required to see the job through. People often come for help when they know they want or need something, but do not know how to do it or get it. They are prevaricating, procrastinating and becoming irritated because of their unmet need, but do not know how to address it. By helping them find the information and skills they need, we can help people motivate themselves to move over the threshold into the unknown and deliver for themselves.

Listening to their language can give us some helpful pointers. Their modal operators, the words that drive their activities, can indicate to us an order in which to direct them. Modal operators come in many forms. The significant ones in this context are *necessity*: "I need to do . . ." *possibility*: "I could do . . ." and *desire*: "I want to do . . ." These will appear in any order as people present their predicament. It can help motivation to focus on the 'need to' statements, and also to reframe the 'wants' and 'coulds' into 'needs' too.

What needs to happen to make a 'want' or 'could' into a 'need'? Sometimes it is just the passage of time: placing a time constraint can increase the sense of urgency, and get people moving. Once action has been taken and a course or direction embarked upon, it is much easier to develop the sense of commitment necessary to see it through.

Asking good questions is an important life skill in any context, including The Consultation. Having the patient ask themselves: "What is in it for me?" is a good way of addressing them to their values and beliefs and stimulating some emotion around their goals. If you want to help someone adapt and change, stimulate some emotion. Make them care and you will motivate them into action.

Summary

In a ten-minute consultation there is always the opportunity to help the patient build their motivation to take responsibility for their health and care. One of the prime professional responsibilities of the doctor is to create a supportive and sustained environment where they can do this. Listening to how the patient presents their predicament can give many useful cues to how best to offer them the help they need to get their state right and get on with the job in hand. The more closely the goal is aligned with their core values, the easier they are going to find it to make progress. This in turn builds motivation to continue.

The best motivator ultimately is taking action. As Nike say: "Just do it."

References

Festinger L. (1957) *A Theory of Cognitive Dissonance* Stanford University Press CA USA
ISBN 978-0804709118

CHAPTER 7 - Taking Action

"The problem is never the problem. It is only a symptom of something much deeper. Coping is the problem."

Virginia Satir

"It is natural forces within us that are the true healers of disease."

Hippocrates

This chapter brings together all that has gone before. It is a collection of ideas to refer to when preparing to consult, and particularly if consulting is not going too well. I have opened with two quotations that draw attention to the doctor's essential role when consulting. This is to approach the consultation in a state of curiosity, with the awareness that there is always more to any situation than meets the eye. Equally important is the knowledge that the patient very often has the resources within or available to them, to address whatever needs dealing with.

I am not seeking to suggest that this awareness is a substitute for appropriate conventional medical intervention, but rather, if we limit ourselves to that, we are only doing, at best, a very partial job. In the time constraints of contemporary General Practice, the work is inevitably broken up into small, bite-sized pieces, but an awareness of how each interaction contributes to a much greater overall mutual strategy can only help towards the generation of the most satisfactory outcomes in any given set of circumstances.

I started with discussions of the importance of state, both the doctor's and the patient's. Awareness of this enables the swift achievement of rapport. Without these the likelihood of a good outcome to a consultation, or any other intervention, is very poor. This was followed by discussion of the identification of hope. The generation of congruent and resourced goals rooted in the patient's values follows. Consideration is then given to how best to help patients find hope and motivate themselves to work on delivering their goals.

This chapter addresses itself to optimising the interaction between the doctor and the patient in the consultation, and the relationship that results from this: the factor identified by Hippocrates as the essential agent of change in the work; the factor that enables the patient to access the Healer Within. The essence of this is good communication. We cannot *not* communicate, so it makes sense to make sure that we communicate well. This invariably starts with listening and observing optimally. This takes time, but not necessarily a lot. Listening, watching, and calibrating both the patient's and our own emotions and responses at the beginning of a consultation determine how effectively we conduct the remainder of it. It also enables us to convey the message to the patient that we are interested in them and their situation, that we believe they have the resources to address whatever it is they need to address, and that we will provide the professional sponsorship they need as they move on.

Taking action

At no point have we touched on the content of what the patient brings. It is very easy to get side-tracked by the minutiae of the patient's account of their woes and neglect the bigger picture. We can be so busy counting the beans that we forget to taste the stew.

I have sought to identify the principles of the approach I have generated for myself over 38 years that have helped me keep at least a part of my attention on the holistic context of the work and which has made consulting with patients such an enjoyable and satisfying aspect of my career. The problem the patient presents is never the fundamental problem for the doctor. Identifying how the patient is doing the problem and helping them make the changes and adjustments they need to achieve their desired results is the essence of the doctor's role. The Latin root of the word 'doctor' is 'teacher'. One of the doctor's duties to the patient is as an educator.

The vast majority of patients who present in General Practice are not broken and do not need fixing. It is, of course, crucial that the doctor spots the ones who do need some fixing-type intervention and gets on with providing or arranging this. At the same time, there is always the opportunity for the educational role too. Our job is to set the environment as well as we can for the patient to best address their issues: to help them create for themselves the contexts and processes which are going to serve them best. While it is often helpful for a patient to gain some insight into how they are contributing to what is happening in their life, this knowledge is not enough to be of significant help to them. It is the meaning that people ascribe to their experience and the values and beliefs that evolve that determine where they place their attention and generate their responses.

This is where the work takes place. Einstein is reputed to have said: "You cannot change something at the level of thinking which created it." Helping people to develop some objectivity about their situation is immensely valuable in helping them motivate themselves to start changing what they can do to help themselves. This is fundamentally at the level of attitude: a metaphor from the science of avionics: the angle of approach. This has to be right for a soft landing. Human beings are meaning-makers. Giving meaning to our experience is very important for building motivation and resilience.

The essential skills that underlie this process have been touched on at several points in the discussions so far. The most important skill set of all is calibration. This means giving full attention to the patient, using every sense available, to build an appreciation of how they are constructing their experience. This insight can then guide us to how and where best to intervene in the patient's experience to help them move along. This awareness also allows us to build rapport quickly: it guides us to communicate with patients on their terms, so they have the best chance of following what is being communicated. This also allows congruence to be maintained, and, more specifically, to spot when either the doctor or the patient is becoming incongruent; when the "yes, but . . ." starts to appear. These points are important and, if ignored, will quickly derail an interaction.

Taking action

Another skill set I wish to highlight is the asking of good questions. These are questions that gently encourage the patient to examine how they are constructing their world and creating their incongruities. This helps give them choice about whether they want to do something about it. Good questions elicit emotions and a 'felt-sense' about experience. As goals emerge, attaching emotions to them brings judgement and values into play and the opportunity to check for congruence and incongruence. A useful short-cut, that is often helpful and efficient, is to ask people what they want, or what they would like to happen, and how they will know when they have got it. If there is something they want to be rid of, rephrasing the questions slightly is all that is required: "What would they like to be rid of? How will they know when it has gone?" As they go inside and start working on answers to these questions, it is important to watch and calibrate for congruence.

When information emerges, further questioning to have them explore what this would do for them, and particularly what this would mean for them, and the effects these changes in them might have on others, will quickly but indirectly bring out their underlying values and beliefs. More information can be gathered by asking what they feel is stopping them, and what resources they feel they need. A further source of motivation can emerge if what will happen if they do not change is also explored. All these questions will elicit the patient's values and beliefs, and direct appropriate responses, as it is at the level of belief that the effective change work takes place. The problem is never the problem, modulating how they are responding to the problem is where effective change is produced. (Satir, 1991)

A bedside manner

To the above mix, I would add that a good sense of humour is essential. Dealing with poor health and emotional and psychological challenges is serious stuff, but it is my view that until people can start to laugh and lighten up a little, when appropriate, it is very difficult for them to shake themselves out of the unresourceful states they find themselves in. Encouraging this requires great sensitivity on the part of the doctor. Do what you do seriously, with great humour.

Our state is very largely a function of where we are placing our focus, our attention. My suggestion is that generally this is best placed in the future. The most useful function of the conscious mind is planning the future. This is often best preceded by some reflection on the experiences of the past and particularly the learnings that have come from those experiences. The conscious mind also has a further useful function; the creation of a positive meeting and holding place for experience, so creativity, learning, growth and constructive change can emerge. The essence of any successful intervention is in helping our patients create desired futures for themselves in their imagination, then accessing the resources necessary to deliver them, and then having them get on with the job. Every situation we meet is unique. Bringing a child-like curiosity to every moment is a very powerful way of maintaining mental flexibility, which is itself vital to learning.

The above can be summed up with the advice to don our 'L' plates when consulting and *Listen* (with an attitude of creative curiosity); *Laugh*; *Look* (to the future); and *Learn*.

Taking action

A good consultation with a patient is a conversation with a purpose. The outcome depends largely on the patient's expectations and their motivation. The setting of mutually-agreed and mutually-congruent goals is essential to even get this far. This raises the issue of permission. The doctor has a huge knowledge-base, a vast range of skills and techniques, and often considerable experience at their disposal. The doctor is in a very powerful position to influence the patient with the suggestions that are made in the consultation. An anxious, distressed and suffering patient is in a very vulnerable and suggestible state. It might be assumed that, because the patient is seeking help, that consent is implied for the doctor to proceed as they think best. At all stages of the consultation it is necessary to maintain a dialogue with the patient to check that they understand how the doctor is interpreting their perceptions of their issues and their requests and is in agreement with whatever is being suggested and the way things are going.

This process has the advantage of being a good way of building and maintaining rapport too, which is essential for any effective change work. The doctor's sensory acuity, the ability to calibrate and check that the consultation is on course, then comes into play, and the flexibility to adjust and adapt as necessary to keep the whole process on track. The doctor needs to be in the optimum learning state: curious, creative, and in touch with all the necessary resources, internal and external. The process outlined above unfolds best in the context of the attitude of creative curiosity in both the doctor and the patient. The problem is never the problem. The problem is always how the patient is 'doing' their response to the problem. The solution emerges when the patient's patterning is interrupted, and something more useful substituted. At this point some specific discussion about communication will be helpful.

We cannot *not* communicate, and the fact that communication is constantly taking place both internally in the participants and externally between them is implicit in all that has been presented thus far. Consulting is most effective if the communication from the doctor to the patient is clear and efficient. This does not mean it always has to be direct: information communicated indirectly is often much more effective than direct commands and instruction (paraphrasing Heraclitus). These do have their place of course. Compliance is likely to be best if the patient receives suggestions both directly and indirectly. Telling is not teaching. It is often necessary to repeat instructions several times and present them in several different ways (oral, written, visual, online etc.). Again, calibration is key: checking that the patient has received, understood, and assimilated the necessary information and instructions and is motivated and determined to deliver is a constant and continual part of the doctor-patient relationship. This can then be supplemented by appropriate anecdotes, including accounts that describe how other patients have prevailed in similar circumstances.

Change is inevitable. Part of our role as doctors is to help catalyse desired change in and for our patients; to help them adjust and adapt to their changing circumstances, and, where possible, to educate and empower them to influence these processes. The body-mind has built in processes for resilience and is designed to heal and restore function if given the appropriate resources and opportunities to do so.

Taking action

In clinical practice change often has to start at the level of belief. I have already stressed the importance of identifying and building hope and motivation and focusing on desired outcomes. Belief is essentially a feeling and is thus closely associated with values. Beliefs are not held in the conscious mind but can be brought into conscious awareness by the feelings they produce. In this context, thinking in terms of cause and effect is therefore of limited value: by the time a person is aware of a feeling, the underlying belief-set is already active. In change work it is helpful to follow the model described by Victor Frankl (the founder of Logotherapy) and think in terms of stimulus and response. A given stimulus (such as a thought), will produce an associated, habitually-patterned response. If the doctor can help the patient to be aware of this and interrupt the pattern, they can then explore other options and start voluntarily to modify their thoughts, feelings and behaviours, and break the neuro-muscular lock which has held them in their habitual responses. Victor Frankl said: "Between stimulus and response there is a space. In that space is our power to choose our response. In our response lies our growth and our freedom." This reflects Epicetus (Epicetus, 135 AD) "In the moment we have control of nothing except our own state. It is not what happens to us, but how we react to it that matters".

Human beings are meaning-making machines. Once the basic instincts of safety and survival have been addressed, people like to make sense of their experience. Another very fundamental instinct is familiarity. We like to analyse our experience and compare it to what we already know to see how it fits in. If it does, we have congruence and feel comfortable. If it does not, we feel uncomfortable and this motivates us to change. This is the basis of learning. I discussed Festinger's cognitive dissonance in

Chapter 6 when discussing motivation. This is the discomfort experienced when a core belief is challenged. It is typically the feeling we experience when our beliefs and behaviours do not match or are contradictory. We do not tolerate it long: either belief changes to adapt to behaviour or our behaviour adapts to our belief. This is different to anger, which is the emotion felt when a core value is challenged.

Calibration is again key here, both of our own responses and those of our patients. Spotting this cognitive dissonance gives us the opportunity for timely intervention. In Chapter 2, when discussing rapport, I discussed how the 'language' (words and physiology) a patient is using, gives many clues to how they are constructing their experience. We can then use this awareness to help them reframe their perceptions in subtle ways that allow and facilitate the desired change.

There are many excellent specific language techniques that can be used at this point which are beyond the scope of this short book. The interested reader will find much to help them in the linguistic models developed by Richard Bandler and John Grinder, based on Chomsky's Transformational Grammar (Bandler and Grinder, 1979). They coined the term Neuro-Linguistic Programming for their work and it has influenced thinking, learning and progress in many diverse fields over the last 40 years. The rudiments can be found in their early books (Bandler and Grinder, 1975). These techniques cannot, however be adequately learned from books. They are experiential and are best studied under the tutelage of experienced and appropriately-trained teachers. NLP is essentially the modelling of excellence. It can be applied in any field and leads to an attitude and effective methodology, specific to the need addressed. Having said that, I will offer a brief overview of how I

Taking action

have brought my learning in this field to bear in my professional work.

In the context of the General Practice consultation, the pre-supposition is that *dis-ease* is occurring because the body and the mind are out of rapport with each other. The work is in re-establishing this communication: identifying how the patient is doing what they are doing, rather than what they are doing: the patterns and processing of what is happening, rather than the content. A further pre-supposition is that all behaviour is purposeful. At some, unconscious level, there is a positive intent to what is happening. This approach requires establishing a co-operative relationship between all the parts of a patient's personality to generate ecologically-sound outcomes that meet their needs and no longer require the unwanted behaviour, symptoms or disease. I have mentioned the importance of asking good questions. In this approach the fundamental question for the doctor is: "How are they doing that?". When the pattern has been identified, the challenge is to interrupt the patterning long enough to allow for the emergence of congruent alternatives. This is best done subtly by means of open questions that direct the patient towards their objectives.

Goal-setting and starting with the end in mind can be simply addressed by asking: "What do you want?" and calibrating the response for congruence. This can then be followed up by the equally important question of: "How will you know when you have got it?". This question seeks to specify what the senses will be perceiving when the desired goal is reached, and also what emotions will be felt. There is no retrospection in this approach. It is based on three pre-suppositions: The best thing about the past is that it is over; there is only ever now; and we are working with current neurological processing.

Summary

What I suggest we are aiming for in the consultation is the optimum learning state in ourselves and our patients: a state of creative curiosity which allows for analysis and permits intuitions and internal and external resources in both doctor and patient to produce new patterns. Fundamental to this is our intention congruently to help, sponsor and support our patients as they find their ways through their lives and experiences. This invariably means, for both doctor and patient, exploring the sweet spot between what is already known and familiar, and the unfamiliar and therefore threatening unknown. This requires courage and the deployment of considerable skill and expertise, including calibration, building and maintaining congruence and rapport, asking better questions and continually questioning the answers that emerge. All this needs to be done with judicious doses of humour at appropriate times. Until people can laugh, it is very difficult for them to change. Do what you do seriously, with great humour. This is no place for hubris. The work must be approached with humility if it is to be successful. An open, child-like mind, tempered with some scepticism is essential to optimise the chances of success. When consulting with our patients we need to be wearing our 'L'-plates: Listen, Laugh, Look to the future and Learn.

References

Satir V. (1991): *The Patterns of her Magic*.

Steve Andreas Real People Press

ISBN0-911226-38-9

Taking action

Bandler R. and Grinder J. (1979) *Frogs Into Princes* 1979 Richard Bandler and John Grinder   Real People Press ISBN 0-911226-19-2

Bandler R. and Grinder J. (1975 and 1976) *The Structure of Magic 1 and 2* Science and Behaviour Books (1975) ISBN 08314-0044-7 (1976) ISBN 08314-0049-8

A bedside manner

CHAPTER 8 - Reflecting and Learning

At the beginning of this book I made the point that the meaning of the word 'doctor' is 'teacher', and that an important part of the doctor's work is educational. This process applies equally to both doctor and patient. Education is a cyclical process. Experience occurs and then a process of reflection is necessary to review what has happened, what has gone well and what might have been different. This then creates an opportunity for some planning and preparation. The cycle can then be repeated indefinitely. The patient will certainly be looking for some feedback from the doctor in this reflective process. There will also be plenty of feedback from the patient to the doctor. Although this may be less explicit, it will be perfectly apparent if the doctor is observant and curious. It is a feature of adult learners that they look for feedback on their performance and are highly sensitive to it. One of the many skills of doctors is the development of a protective second-skin so that they can retain some objectivity about their own performance, learn from experience and make the necessary adjustments while still protecting and preserving their own integrity and health.

Calibration has come up repeatedly throughout this work and is here again now. Paying attention throughout the consultation, checking on comprehension, compliance and progress and sharing these observations with the patient all maintain rapport, keep the process on course, and allow for the planning of the next stage. While paying attention in the moment is essential, it is also vital to have set the course in advance. This is done by placing the focus of our attention in the future and making plans. This is the most useful function of the conscious mind. The conscious mind observes what the neurology has already set in place. The order is: things happen, we become aware of them and then respond. Essentially all we have to work with is the neurology active in the present moment: our state. The work is in accessing the right state in ourselves for the situation, then placing the focus externally and into the future, and taking appropriate action. This resembles deploying a guided missile: the process is load the state, fire, then direct to the target, which may well be moving so constant calibration and adjustment are required.

This requires constant vigilance and regular review. The more we can educate our patients to take this on, the better for all concerned. The skills of goal-setting, building rapport both with ourselves (body and mind) and externally with others and our environment, and paying attention to what is happening so we can maintain and appropriately and flexibly adjust our state and behaviour can all be taught, learned, practised and mastered. Regular reflection is essential for this learning to take place, and is an important part of following up and reviewing patients. This educational process contributes significantly to enhancing resilience: the ability to withstand stress. When we reflect, we can give meaning to our experience, even in adversity. In this way we can learn from our experience, become stronger and cope better. Just knowing is not enough. In the medical context, the science (Greek: *knowing, knowledge*) is not enough. Insight is also insufficient on its own. It is the meaning that we ascribe to our experience and the values and beliefs that evolve from this that determine where we place our attention and generate our response. This is where the work takes place. To paraphrase

Reflecting and learning

Einstein, we cannot change something at the level of thinking that created it. We have to create a place beyond simple, rational, logical explanation, where we can experience our response to our predicament and allow access to resources from beyond the conscious domain to formulate our responses. The best insights, ideas and learnings often emerge after we have ceased grappling consciously with an issue and allowed the unconscious mind to process it while the conscious mind is asleep.

This is not to say that there is not a place for some structured, cognitive work. This is often the apparent content of the consultation. The Japanese practice of Kaizen, continuous improvement, provides a convenient frame for this. Again, we are seeking to ask good questions: "What is going well?". This sets a positive frame of mind but it is important not to dwell too long here. "What could be done differently?" is a question worth spending time on. Formulating options and thinking them through so the best one can be selected is worth the extra effort. Often, options that give results in the short-term may produce more and greater problems down the road, so giving some consideration to potential medium and long-term outcomes is always time well spent. It is important then to take a decision and move on with the next cycle.

Regular review also allows time for feedback: objective opinion from a trusted source is invaluable. This needs to be structured and controlled, factually-based, and be motivational and developmental. If not, there is a danger that it will turn into criticism. Criticism has no place in an educational process. It is a crude form of bullying and manipulation. It is, however, an excellent way of breaking constructive rapport, if this is ever necessary.

Dr Arthur Hibble, the former Director of our regional GP training scheme, taught that when teaching registrars, feedback should be owned, constructive, regular, specific, balanced and clear. These are excellent guidelines for a teacher to follow, and are as applicable in the GP consultation as they are in the tutorial. Indeed, the two processes are much the same.

Owned: the consultation is the patient's. One of the reasons for building and maintaining rapport is for the patient to take ownership of the process. If they feel that what is emerging is their idea, or at least rooted in their ideas, they are far more likely to be compliant with whatever strategy emerges.

Constructive: whatever emerges builds towards pre-agreed, congruent goals.

Regular: adult learners generally like feedback that they are on the right track, and appreciation for what has already been achieved. This is most effective if provided on a fairly regular basis, although the intervals can be wide.

Specific: The more detailed and specific the feedback is, the more likely it is to be understood and built on.

Balanced: The Kaizen process allows time to both appreciate the successes and drive the necessary changes.

Clear: the use of simple, clean language which the patient himself uses and understands is the best way of ensuring compression and compliance. This includes an appreciation of their preferred representational systems, as discussed in Chapter 2 on rapport.

Reflecting and learning

A further model for reflection I have used in training GPs and with coaching patients is based on a technique known as ALOBA (Silverman JD, Kurtz SM and Draper J, 1996): agenda-led, outcome-based analysis. My understanding is that the structure is essentially a combination of Kaizen with an outcome-focus added, generating alternatives. It is similar to the structured questions suggested in the previous chapter but starting with some retrospection. The questions might follow a pattern something like this:

- What were we seeking to achieve?
- How well did we do it?
- What next?
- What is already helping?
- What do we need?
- How will we know?

These are all open questions. The doctor is not making any suggestions regarding content in these exchanges. The doctor provides the framework and the process and the patient provides the content. This is very clean work that highly respects the patient's autonomy and provides a supportive environment in which they can use their creativity to generate what they want for themselves.

Finally, I remember Roger Callahan, who developed Thought Field Therapy, saying that anyone who claims 100% success for any line of management has not treated enough people. He was undoubtedly a genius, but his work was performed and presented with great humility. It is possible to apply all the principles I have outlined in these pages and the patient not achieve their desired outcomes. This is inevitable. It is not failure: this is seldom a useful frame. It is feedback and should be treated as such. There are always lessons to be learned. After appropriate reflection, the learning can be taken from these experiences: we learn much more from them than we do from our successes. This is where we can do a great service to our patients, in our role as coach and mentor. Shortly after his retirement from competitive professional tennis, Boris Becker, when asked about his formula for success replied that it was to set goals congruently, be determined, have humility, ask and listen. The objectivity of an authoritative, reliable and trusted observer is invaluable. It behoves us to be this for our patients and our students.

References

Silverman JD, Kurtz SM and Draper J (1996) - *The Cambridge-Calgary approach to communication skills teaching. Agenda led outcome-based analysis of the consultation.* Educ Gen Pract 7:288-99

CHAPTER 9 - Resistance

Finally, some thoughts about how to meet most effectively with resistance in the consultation; when things are not running smoothly. In other words: what to do when it is not working.

State and rapport

Somewhat predictably, the first port of call is to review your state. If any sort of rapport has been established with your patient, how you are feeling is likely to be a reflection of how they are feeling. By the same token, if you are paying attention and calibrating your state, when the patient struggles, if you optimise your state and reinforce and increase rapport, it is highly likely that the patient's state will also improve. Sometimes this is all that is required. As the patient improves their state, so they approach 'flow' and have best access to their problem-solving skills. In this state, solutions can start to emerge and 'problems' disappear. Remember, it is almost always not the problem that is the problem, but rather, how the patient is doing the problem that requires adaptation. As we have seen, states can easily be modulated by altering physiology, language and redirecting focus. Once the state of all parties has been re-optimised and a better feeling of rapport established, other areas to explore are:

Congruence

It is very common to hear: "Yes, but . . ." We may think we have established good states and rapport, and negotiated and set good goals, but we are working in an ever-changing environment.

What appeared congruent and compelling yesterday may have lost its allure today. Awareness, calibration and flexibility are key. Goal-setting and reviewing and the building of hope and motivation need to be constantly updated. The "yes . . . but" response tells us congruence had been lost, and we need to go back to where the process broke down and re-establish rapport. From this point we can get back on track for a goal which may well have changed, or be in need of re-framing and approaching in a different way.

Safety and fear

One of the most fundamental human instincts is familiarity. It takes a lot of determination and motivation to step out of the comfort-zone and into the unknown. Change will only occur when the alternative is more desirable than the status-quo. It has to be a lot more desirable for people to step over the threshold and go for it. It helps if the status-quo is becoming increasingly undesirable and uncomfortable too. If this appears to be the case, then it is worth revisiting motivation. People need to be fully motivated and determined to deliver the outcomes they have chosen.

Limiting beliefs

Effective and lasting change will only occur if the patient wants it and is prepared to take responsibility for doing whatever is necessary to deliver it, and be accountable for whatever the outcome. Particularly, they have to be able to answer to themselves; wherever they go they take themselves with them; they are the only constant presence in their lives. If they do not believe that the person they are asking for help is the right person, or do not believe that they have the competence to deliver the outcomes they have identified for themselves, the chances of success are very slim. If this is the case then motivation needs to be revisited. Possibly goals also need to reviewed and some more congruent ones identified. Some new skills, knowledge or attitudes may need to be developed. Other limiting beliefs often encountered include a strong sense of responsibility for others, and feelings of guilt and possibly shame. If the patient does achieve the changes, what might the effect be on others in their life?

This brings us back to reconsideration of the ecology frame in the goal-setting. The goals may need reviewing. Another limiting belief that often arises is the illusion of control. This can be the perception that someone or something is seeking to control them, or conversely, that they are unable to control someone or something else. Whatever the case, the truth is that we have very little, if any, control of events or other people's thoughts, feelings or behaviour, or our own in the instant for that matter. This is why reflection is so important. Things happen, internally and externally, and we have to respond to them. We have very little control over what goes on. We do have a choice about our responses. Our ability to make better choices can be significantly improved by awareness and practice.

When things are not running to plan, it is also important to be vigilant for dissociation. The patient will very often have no idea why they are unable to get started or continue along on a path. Very often a part of them to which they have no conscious access is at work, apparently obstructing progress. The key here is to be aware that whatever is happening, the part of them that is controlling it has a positive intention for the patient. The 'resistance' or 'problem' is this unconscious part seeking recognition and human contact. Meeting this with curiosity, and seeking to understand what values are at work may well permit some constructive reframing of what is happening so that new goals and strategies can emerge. The point is that it is not going to help to meet resistance with resistance. All that will do is escalate the impasse. There is an energy at work and it is much easier to redirect a stream than it is to dam it up. The solution to the problem is very often to be found in the resistance. Whatever is happening has a positive intention for the person and whatever solutions emerge need to maintain this benefit. This is commonly the case when tension, emotional strain and unresolved conflicts are part of the picture. Everything that is happening is happening for a feeling, for the meeting of a value.

Patients are often patients because of where they are directing their focus of attention. This may be internally and they perceive themselves as the victims rather than the heroes of their stories, or externally where they are heading for incongruent goals or fleeing from non-existent threats.

In these circumstances some constructive re-framing can be very helpful. Patients can feel a sense of liberation when they realise that their thoughts are just that; thoughts. They are not the 'truth', just thoughts: some neuro-biological activity in their mind. A belief is essentially a feeling of certainty about a thought. Once people realise that these thoughts are theirs and they can decide what to think and focus on and what to let pass, then they can allow intrusive thoughts to move on through without engaging with them, and deliberately aim the focus of their thoughts where they will gain the most: the future, and how they

Resistance

will be when they no longer have the problems they have in the present. They do not have to believe everything they think.

It is important not to meet resistance with resistance, but to welcome it with openness and a creative curiosity: a wish to understand. If you do not resist resistance it loses its power. If you give them long enough, patients will tell you what the problem is. If you give them a bit longer, they will reveal what needs to happen.

A bedside manner

CHAPTER 10 - Summary

So that is it. I have broken the process of the consultation into eight chunks for the purposes of illustration and discussion. In reality, they are not discrete steps but all part of a continuum. When consulting is running smoothly it is usually because these boxes are being ticked. When things start to go awry, awareness of these factors will help to identify where some adjustment is likely to pay dividends.

The steps are:

1.   Accessing your optimum state: creative curiosity with an empty, engaged and open mind.

2.   Building rapport: calibrating.

3.   Helping the patient to access their optimum state: summoning Hippocrates' "Healer Within".

4.   Installing hope.

5.   Setting congruent goals.

6.   Building motivation.

7.   Taking action.

8.   Reflecting and learning.

Steps 1 to 3 need to be done first and in that order. After that, the order in which I have presented them is a good working model but does not need to be slavishly adhered to. Steps 4 to 8 apply equally to the clinician as to the patient.

This structure is applicable to any situation where individuals are seeking help with something that they are struggling to address on their own. I have referred very little to the content of the consultation. The patient provides this initially, with the doctor judiciously adding their knowledge and skills at the appropriate points. The patient presents their narrative of their experience and I suggest it is the doctor's role to be as supportive of this where appropriate and also, at times, directive. This is often done subtly. Joseph Campbell (Campbell, 1949) described the Hero's Journey. An important part of our role is that of mentor and teacher; helping our patient access the strength and drive to enter this Hero mode and staying with it, rather than sinking into impotent and blaming Victimhood. Diagnosis, therapeutics, teamwork and onward referral are all fundamental to a doctor's work. There is much else to be done in addition to these.

A fundamental belief that has underlined all my professional practice is that 'doctor' means 'teacher'. Throughout my career I have sought to identify learning needs as well as therapeutic and interventional ones. This awareness includes myself. Every situation we encounter is unique and both doctor and patient are having new learning needs generated all the time. This parallel processing has been one of the underlying themes of this book. Whatever is happening to and for the patient has an effect on the doctor too. The participant's awareness of this parallel processing and their responses to it are what creates the flow and the musicality of the successful consultation. Not paying attention, or

Summary

paying attention but not responding and moving congruently with the unfolding situation is what generates poor outcomes. Once medically diagnosable and treatable 'illness' has been identified and appropriately addressed, the tuned-in doctor can do much to help the patient address their learning needs too, and redirect their energy into congruent, ecologically-sound goals. This paradigm shift for the doctor, the doctor as teacher rather than therapist, allows other levels of parallel processing to be running simultaneously: learning and healing. The keys to this are constant and accurate calibration of self and patient, the formulation of good questions, and then the sensitive questioning of the answers which emerge so the underlying processing can be identified and made available to the patient for them to adapt. I see the doctor's role in this as being like the Second in the corner in the boxing ring: the consultation presents the opportunity for some reflection and brief intervention, then the warrior is sent back out into the fray.

There are a number of themes that run through these chapters. I have discussed the parallel processing which is occurring in the paragraphs above. Related to this is the importance of state, and the fact that states are contagious. We pick them up from the patient and they pick ours up. The better the rapport that has been established, the more efficiently this happens.

A third theme is the phenomenon of the body keeping the score. Our conscious thoughts occur very late in the processing. Things happen within us and in our environment. Our senses detect what is happening and unconsciously process the information before the parts of the brain involved in cognition have any access to the processed material. The body communicates with feelings and emotions, it does not have spoken language. The words we use to describe our experience are a response to the very limited information that reaches the cognitive parts of the brain. This is why calibration is so important. The patient's physiology is giving us a lot of information all the time that they have no conscious awareness of. Responding appropriately to this is essential.

The most basic skill to all this work is awareness. Mindfulness is an ancient practice that is in essence the practice on conscious awareness (Hanh, 1975). Over the last 43 years, since the publishing in 1975 of *The Miracle of Mindfulness* by Thich Nhat Hanh, the Western world has become increasingly aware of just how powerful and globally-helpful this practice is. It is a skill which can be practised and developed. It is the absence of a mindful approach to life that leads to much of the suffering that presents to a GP. There is great wisdom in awareness, and introducing mindful practice into their daily lives is something we can usefully teach our patients. Not least this can help them become aware of the destructive power of taking a single position on any issue as this potentially robs them of the ability to live fulfilled lives in every moment. Alfred Korzybski (Korzybski, 1958) said: "whatever you think it is, it is not." Every situation we find ourselves in is just one of an infinite range of possibilities that happens to fit the moment. If it works that is fine. Carry on and learn and grow. If it is not working then this is an opportunity to change. The effective changes are subtle, internal adaptations of attitude: micro-movements. Not seismic external abreactive change. This usually leads to more problems. When someone is stuck in suffering invariably it is because a part has lost contact with the whole and is being held in isolation, without the musicality of creative flow. The work is not in resisting this part and seeking to 'treat' it, but rather welcoming it in and listening

Summary

from a centred, open, subtly aware, resourced and compassionately holding place to the message it is seeking to convey: the need that is seeking expression. What we are seeking is the integrating of the isolated part with the collective wisdom of the whole and restoring the musicality of generative flow. Nice work if you can get it.

We can do this simply by asking good questions, starting with: "How do you do that?"

References

Campbell. J (1949) *The Hero with 1000 Faces*. New World Library ISBN 978-1-57731-593-3

Korzybski A. (1958) *Science and Sanity: An Introduction to Non-Aristotelian Systems and General Semantics*

Hanh T. (2008) *The Miracle of Mindfulness* Rider Books, London, UK

ISBN 978-1-84-604106-8

A bedside manner

INDEX

Index

Printed in Poland
by Amazon Fulfillment
Poland Sp. z o.o., Wrocław

62040195R00060